Disclaimer Notice:

Please note the information contained within this document is for educational and entertainment purposes only. All effort has been executed to present accurate, up to date, and reliable, complete information. No warranties of any kind are declared or implied. Readers acknowledge that the author is not engaging in the rendering of legal, financial, medical or professional advice. The content within this book has been derived from various sources. Please consult a licensed professional before attempting any techniques outlined in this book.

By reading this document, the reader agrees that under no circumstances is the author responsible for any losses, direct or indirect, which are incurred as a result of the use of information contained within this document, including, but not limited to, errors, omissions, or inaccuracies.

Table of Content

Introduction

Thank you for purchasing **Healthy Ketogenic Diet Cookbook: A Completet Guide With Healthy and Easy Keto Diet Recipes To Weight Loss, Burn Fat And Live Better**

The ketogenic diet began as a low-carbohydrate dietary plan aimed at reducing seizures in patients who did not respond to medication, especially in children. Very low carbohydrate diets have been used since the 1920s for this very purpose.

Since the sixties, these diets have been widely used for the treatment of obesity, but also in the presence of other pathological conditions such as diabetes, polycystic ovary syndrome, acne: it was in fact observed that, in addition to acting on convulsions, they produced positive effects on body fat, blood sugar, cholesterol and hunger levels.

The ketogenic diet has, therefore, increasingly established itself as a diet to lose weight, which exploits the consequences for the body of the reduction of carbohydrates and the increased consumption of fats, not for therapeutic purposes, but to stimulate weight loss.

BREAKFAST

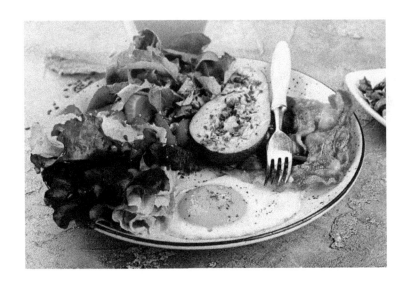

Pork Rind Waffles

Preparation Time: 5 minutes

Cooking Time: 10 minutes

Servings: 4

Ingredients:

*   4 large eggs

*   4 ounces cream cheese, at room temperature

*   1 teaspoon erythritol

*   2 teaspoons ground cinnamon

*   2 teaspoons vanilla extract

*   1½ teaspoons baking powder

*   4 tablespoons coconut flour

*   8 tablespoons ground pork rinds (ground in a food processor), divided

*   Nonstick cooking spray

Directions:

1.   Heat the waffle iron.

2.   In the food processor, combine the eggs, cream cheese, erythritol, cinnamon, vanilla, baking powder, coconut flour,

and 6 tablespoons of ground pork rinds. Thoroughly combine until you have a smooth consistency.

3.   Spray the waffle iron with cooking spray and add ¼ to ½ cup of batter to it, depending on the size of your waffle iron. Sprinkle ½ tablespoon of ground pork rinds on top of each waffle, close, and cook until golden brown and crispy.

Nutrition: Calories: 248 Total Fat: 17g Protein: 12g Total Carbs: 10g Fiber: 6g Net Carbs: 4g

Cheesy Thyme Waffles

Preparation Time: 5 minutes

Cooking Time: 10 minutes

Servings: 2

Ingredients:

- ½ cup mozzarella cheese, finely shredded

- ¼ cup Parmesan cheese

- ¼ large head cauliflower

- ½ cup collard greens

- 1 large egg

- 1 stalk green onion

- ½ tablespoon olive oil

- ½ teaspoon garlic powder

- ¼ teaspoon salt

- ½ tablespoon sesame seed

- 1 teaspoon fresh thyme, chopped

- ¼ teaspoon ground black pepper

Directions:

1.   Put cauliflower, collard greens, spring onion and thyme in a food processor and pulse until smooth.

2.   Put mixture in a bowl and mix in rest of the ingredients.

3.   Heat a waffle iron and transfer the mixture evenly over the griddle.

4.   Cook until a waffle is formed and dish out in a serving platter.

Nutrition: Calories: 144 Carbs: 8.5g Fats: 9.4g Proteins: 9.3g Sodium: 435mg Sugar: 3g

Salmon Burrito

Preparation Time: 6 minutes

Cooking Time: 4 minutes

Servings: 2

Ingredients:

- For base and flavor:

- Chopped chives, a pinch

- Dried cumin and coriander, a pinch

- Chopped rosemary, a pinch

- Salt and pepper to taste

- 2 Eggs, (to form a burrito roll)

- Oil for frying the eggs

- For filling:

- ½ Avocado, (chunks)

- ½ cup Salmon, (cooked/boiled)

- ¼ cup Spinach, (cooked/boiled)

Directions:

1. Pick a pan and warm the oil over medium heat.

2.   Mix the egg in a bowl with salt and pepper.

3.   Combine the chives, rosemary, cumin, and coriander in the beaten egg.

4.   Fry the egg and spread each on a separate plate after cooking.

5.   Place the filling over the eggs spread on the plates; equally divide the avocado, spinach, salmon.

6.   Roll the eggs with filling to form in a burrito and serve.

Nutrition: Calories: 331 Fat: 30 g Fiber: 3 g Carbs: 10 gNet Carbs: 7 g Protein: 11 g

KETO BREAD

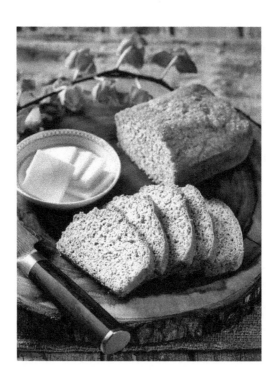

Soft Keto Tortillas

Preparation Time: 10 Minutes

Cooking Time: 35 Minutes

Servings: 6

Ingredients:

- 1 cup coconut flour

- 1/4 teaspoon baking soda

- 1/2 teaspoon salt

- 1/4 cup ground psyllium husk powder

- 1/2 cup avocado oil or olive oil

- 3 large egg whites

- 1 1/2 cup hot water

Directions:

1.   Heat a large cast iron skillet or griddle medium heat.

2.   In a large bowl, sift together the coconut flour, baking soda and salt. Whisk in the psyllium husk.

3.   Drizzle in the oil slowly as you stir the mix, it will become moist and crumbly. Fold in the egg whites.

4.   Mix in the hot water half cup at a time, making sure it's thoroughly mixed in before adding more water. Combine until the dough looks and feels like moist play-doh.

5.   Shape 12 even-sized balls. Flatten the balls between parchment paper on a tortilla press or use a 6" pot and press them down.

6.   Cook 2 tortillas at a time on the large griddle by lying flat on the hot, dry cast iron and toasting 3 minutes a side, flipping once. Set aside until all the tortillas are done.

Nutrition: Calories 250 Fat 21g Protein 6g Carbohydrates 1.7g Fiber 15g

Cheddar Crackers

Preparation Time: 10 minutes

Cooking Time: 55 minutes

Servings: 8

Ingredients:

- 4 Tbsp. unsalted butter, softened slightly

- 1 egg white

- 1/4 tsp. salt

- 1 cup plus 2 Tbsp. almond flour

- 1 tsp. minced fresh thyme

- 1 cup shredded sharp white cheddar cheese

Directions:

1. Preheat the oven to 300F.

2. Using a bowl, beat together the butter, egg white, and salt.

3. Stir in the almond flour, and thyme and then the cheddar until mixed.

4.   Move the dough out between two pieces of parchment paper to a rectangle.

5.   Peel off the top parchment paper and place the dough with the bottom parchment paper on a sheet pan.

6.   Cut the dough into crackers with a pizza cutter.

7.   Bake until golden, about 45 to 55 minutes, rotating the tray once halfway through.

8.   Cool and serve.

Nutrition: Calories: 200 Fat: 18g Carb: 4g Protein: 7g

Cloud Bread

Preparation Time: 13 minutes

Cooking time: 50 minutes

Servings: 10

Ingredients

- 3 large eggs

- 1/4 teaspoon cream of tartar

- 3 ounces cream cheese, softened slightly

- 1 tablespoon heavy whipping cream

- 1/2 teaspoon apple cider vinegar

- 3 drops liquid stevia

- 1/4 cup unflavored whey protein powder

- 3/4 teaspoon psyllium husk powder

- 1/8 teaspoon salt

- 1/8 teaspoon baking powder

Directions:

1. Preheat the oven to 300F.

2. Merge the cream of tartar to the bowl with the egg whites.

3. Attach the cream cheese, cream, vinegar, and liquid stevia to the bowl.

4. Spoon 3 tablespoons batter onto the center of one quadrant of the prepared baking sheet to make a circle; make three more circles in each quadrant of the tray. Repeat with remaining batter on the second prepared baking sheet.

5. Bake until the bread is golden, about 15–20 minutes, rotating the trays once halfway through.

6. Cool the bread on the trays, and then remove each with a thin metal spatula.

Nutrition: Calories 254 Total Fat 11 g Protein 13 g Fiber 2 g Carbohydrates 2.9 g

Press-In Savory Crust

Preparation Time: 5 minutes

Cooking time: 1 hour

Servings: 8

Ingredients

- 11/2 cups plus 1 tablespoon almond flour

- 1/2 teaspoon Italian herb seasoning

- 1/2 teaspoon garlic powder

- 1/2 teaspoon salt

- 1/4 teaspoon black pepper

- 5 tablespoons butter,

Directions:

1. In a medium bowl, stir the almond flour, Italian herb seasoning, garlic powder, salt, and black pepper into the butter until well combined (it will be a bit crumbly).

2. Use this crust to make your favorite quiche or savory pie recipe.

Nutrition: Calories 143 Total Fat 9 g Protein 11 g Fiber 4 g Carbohydrates 4 g

Keto French Toast

Preparation Time: 5 Minutes

Cooking Time: 3 Minutes

Servings: 2

Ingredients:

- Mug bread:

- 1 teaspoon butter

- 2 tablespoons almond flour

- 2 tablespoons coconut flour

- 1 1/2 teaspoon baking powder

- 1 pinch salt

- 2 eggs

- 2 tablespoons heavy whipping cream

- Batter:

- 2 eggs

- 2 tablespoons heavy whipping cream

- 1/2 teaspoon ground cinnamon

- 1 pinch of salt

- 2 tablespoons butter

Directions::

1.   Grease a large mug or glass dish with a flat bottom with butter.

2.   Mix all the dry ingredients together in the mug with a fork or spoon. Crack in the egg and stir in the cream. Combine until smooth and make sure there are no lumps.

3.   Microwave on high (approximately 700 watts) for 2 minutes. Check if the bread is done in the middle – if not, microwave for another 15-30 seconds.

4.   Let it cool and remove from the mug. Slice in half.

5.   In a bowl or deep plate, whisk together the eggs, cream and cinnamon with a pinch of salt. Pour over the bread slices and allow it to soak. Turn it around a few times so the bread slices absorb as much of the egg mixture as possible.

6.   Fry in plenty of butter and serve immediately.

Nutrition: Calories 277 Fat 23g Protein 15g Carbs 4g

Seed And Nut Bread

Preparation Time: 13 minutes

Cooking time: 50 minutes

Servings: 10

Ingredients

- 3 large eggs

- 1/4 cup avocado oil

- 1 teaspoon psyllium husk powder

- 1 teaspoon apple cider vinegar

- 3/4 teaspoon salt

- 5 drops liquid stevia

- 11/2 cups raw unsalted almonds

- 1/2 cup raw unsalted pepitas

- 1/2 cup raw unsalted sunflower seeds

- 1/2 cup flaxseeds

Directions:

1.   Preheat the oven to 325F.

2.   Pour together the eggs, oil, psyllium husk powder, vinegar, salt, and liquid stevia.

3.   Stir in the almonds, pepitas, sunflower seeds, and flaxseeds until well combined.

4.   Bake until the loaf is golden and feels hard to the touch, about 40 minutes.

5.   Cool, and then slice into 1/4"-thick slices.

Nutrition: Calories 232 Total Fat 12 g Protein 11 g Fiber 1 g Carbohydrates 1.9 g

Sandwich Buns

Preparation Time: 13 minutes

Cooking time: 50 minutes

Servings: 10

Ingredients

- 1/2 teaspoon instant yeast
- 2 teaspoons warm water
- 1/2 cup flour
- 3 tablespoons coconut flour
- 1/2 tablespoon psyllium husk powder
- 1/4 teaspoon plus 1/8 teaspoon salt
- 1/4 teaspoon baking powder
- 1 teaspoon beef gelatin
- 11/2 tablespoons plus 3 tablespoons boiling water, divided
- 1/4 cup egg whites
- 1/2 tablespoon apple cider vinegar
- 3 drops liquid stevia
- 11/2 tablespoons ghee, melted
- 1 teaspoon sesame seeds

Directions:

1.   Preheat the oven to 350F.

2.   Merge the yeast and warm water and stir to combine. Set aside until foamy, about 5–10 minutes.

3.   Pour together the almond flour, coconut flour, psyllium husk powder, salt, and baking powder.

4.   Whisk together the beef gelatin and 11/2 tablespoons boiling water until fully dissolved.

5.   Whisk together the dissolved beef gelatin, yeast mixture, egg whites, vinegar, and liquid stevia.

6.   Add this egg white mixture, melted ghee, and 3 tablespoons boiling water to the dry ingredients in the large bowl, and beat with a handheld electric mixer until it forms a dough.

7.   Bake until the rolls are golden

Nutrition: Calories 145 Total Fat 11 g Protein 10 g Fiber 3 g Carbohydrates 3 g

Keto Cornbread

Preparation Time: 10 Minutes

Cooking Time: 20 Minutes

Servings: 8

Ingredients:

- 1/4 cup coconut flour

- 1/3 cup oat fiber

- 1/3 cup whey protein isolate

- 1 1/2 teaspoon baking powder

- 1/4 teaspoon salt

- 4 oz. butter, melted

- 1/3 cup bacon fat or coconut oil, melted

- 1/4 cup water

- 4 eggs

- 1/4 teaspoon corn extract (optional)

Directions:

1.   Preheat oven to 350F. Place a greased 10-inch (25 cm) cast iron skillet in the oven to heat while you make the cornbread.

2.   Combine all the dry ingredients in a bowl.

3. Add the melted butter, bacon fat, eggs, and water. Beat with a hand mixer. Stir in the corn extract.

4. Pour the cornbread mixture into the hot cast iron skillet and bake for about 18 to 20 minutes or until lightly browned and firm to the touch.

5. Tips!

6. The corn extract is optional, but provides a more authentic, corn-like flavor. If you don't have a cast iron skillet, a pie tin or small oven-proof skillet will work.

7. Whey protein isolates has casein and lactose removed and is not the same as whey protein, which can be highly insulinogenic. Please check the ingredients on whey protein isolate to make sure there are no added sweeteners.

8. Oat fiber is the pure insoluble fiber from the outer husk of the oat. Because it is not digestible, it does not impact blood glucose.

Nutrition: Calories 240 Fat 23g Protein 7g Carbohydrates 5g

All-Purpose Roll-Out Crust For Pies

Preparation Time: 5 minutes

Cooking time: 1 hour

Servings: 8

Ingredients

- 3/4 teaspoon beef gelatin
- 4 teaspoons boiling water
- 1/2 teaspoon apple cider vinegar
- 3 drops liquid stevia
- 1 large egg white
- 11/2 cups almond flour
- 2 tablespoons coconut flour
- 1/4 teaspoon plus 1/8 teaspoon salt
- 1/4 teaspoon psyllium husk powder
- 2 tablespoons chilled unsalted butter, diced
- 3 ounces chilled cream cheese, diced

Directions:

1. Merge the beef gelatin and boiling water and stir to dissolve. Allow to cool a few minutes until lukewarm. Whisk in the vinegar, liquid stevia, and egg white.

2. Pour together the almond flour, coconut flour, salt, and psyllium husk powder.

3. Use a fork to combine the egg white mixture into the dry ingredients, and then cut in the butter and cream cheese until it forms a crumbly dough.

4. Gently press the dough together to form a disk. Wrap in plastic wrap and refrigerate until well chilled, at least 2 hours (or up to three days).

Nutrition: Calories 321 Total Fat 11 g Protein 9 g Fiber 4 g Carbohydrates 2.3 g

Soft Tortillas

Preparation Time: 5 minutes

Cooking time: 1 hour

Servings: 6

Ingredients

- 1 cup egg whites

- 1/4 cup avocado oil

- 1 cup almond flour

- 1/4 cup coconut flour

- 1 tablespoon psyllium husk powder

- 1 teaspoon salt

- 1/2 teaspoon onion powder

- 1/2 teaspoon garlic powder

- 11/2 cups boiling water

Directions:

1. Pour together all ingredients except the boiling water.

2. Add the boiling water and beat until smooth.

3. Heat a medium nonstick skillet over medium to medium-high heat.

4.   Pour 1/4 cup batter onto the heated skillet. Using the measuring cup, quickly spread out the batter as thin as you can without breaking the tortilla, to a circle about 5"–6" in diameter.

5.   Cook until the tortilla is golden, about 2–3 minutes.

6.   Flip, and then cook until golden on the second side, about 1–2 minutes more. Place the tortilla on a plate, and repeat with the remaining batter.

Nutrition: Calories 165 Total Fat 12 g Protein 14 g Fiber 2 g Carbohydrates 1 g

Sweet Vanilla Cream Biscuits

Preparation Time: 5 minutes

Cooking time: 1 hour

Servings: 8

Ingredients

- 1 cup almond flour

- 3 tablespoons powdered erythritol

- 1 teaspoon baking powder

- 1/4 teaspoon salt

- 2 tablespoons chilled unsalted butter, diced

- 2 ounces chilled cream cheese, diced

- 1/2 tablespoon pure vanilla extract

- 1/2 teaspoon pure almond extract

- 10 drops liquid stevia

- 1 large egg, lightly beaten

Directions:

1.   Preheat the oven.

2.   Merge together the almond flour, powdered erythritol, baking powder, and saltUse a fork to mix in the vanilla and almond extracts, liquid stevia, and then the egg.

3.   Cut the dough, and roll each into a ball (their shape doesn't have to be perfect).

4.   Serve warm or at room temperature.

Nutrition: Calories 321 Total Fat 11 g Protein 9 g Fiber 4 g Carbohydrates 2.3 g

KETO PASTA

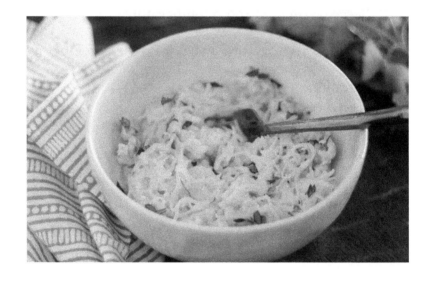

Delicious Sambal Seitan Noodles

Preparation Time: 12 minutes

Cooking Time: 60 minutes

Servings: 4

Ingredients:

- For the shirataki noodles:
- 2 (8 oz.) packs Miracle noodles, garlic and herb
- Salt to season
- For the sambal seitan:
- 1 tbsp. olive oil
- 1 lb. seitan
- 4 garlic cloves, minced
- 1-inch ginger, peeled and grated
- 1 tsp. liquid Erythritol
- 1 tbsp. sugar-free tomato paste
- 2 fresh basil leaves + extra for garnishing
- 2 tbsp. sambal oelek
- 2 tbsp. plain vinegar
- 1 cup water

- 2 tbsp. coconut aminos

- Salt to taste

- 1 tbsp. unsalted butter

Directions:

1. For the shirataki noodles:

2. Bring water to a boil in a over medium heat.

3. Strain the Miracle noodles through a colander and rinse very well under hot running water.

4. Allow proper draining and pour the noodles into the boiling water. Cook for 3 minutes and strain again.

5. Place a dry skillet over medium heat and stir-fry the shirataki noodles until visibly dry, 1 to 2 minutes. Season with salt, plate and set aside.

6. For the seitan sambal:

7. Heat the olive oil and cook in the seitan until brown, 5 minutes.

8. Stir in the garlic, ginger, liquid erythritol and cook for 1 minute.

9.   Add the tomato paste, cook for 2 minutes and mix in the basil, sambal oelek, vinegar, water, coconut aminos, and salt.

10.   Uncover, add the shirataki noodles, butter and mix well into the sauce.

11.   Dish the food, garnish with some basil leaves and serve warm.

Nutrition: Calories: 538 Total Fat: 41.1g Total Carbs: 2g Fiber: 14g Sugar: 5g Protein: 29g

Shrimp Pad Thai With Shirataki Noodles

Preparation Time: 5 minutes

Cooking time: 30 minutes

Servings: 3

Ingredients

* Shirataki fettuccini noodles (2 pkg. - 7 oz. each)

* Medium-sized wild-caught shrimp (18)

* Pastured eggs (2)

* Brain Octane Oil - divided (1.5 tbsp.)

* Coconut aminos (2 tbsp.)

* Lime (1 juiced & divided)

* Cashew butter (1 tsp.)

* Garlic (1 clove)

* Crushed red pepper (.25 tsp.)

* Cilantro (.25 cup)

* Green onions (2)

* Sea salt

* Optional for the Garnish: Cashews - crushed (4)

Directions

1.   Finely mince the garlic and chop the onions.

2.   Prepare the shirataki noodles using the package instructions (rinsing for 15 seconds, boiling for 2 minutes in a pot of water, and draining the noodles. Place them in a dry skillet without oil using the medium heat and "dry roast" them for one minute). Set aside.

3.   In a small mixing container, combine 0.75 of a tablespoon of the Brain Octane Oil, cashew butter, garlic, coconut aminos, 1/2 of the lime juice, and crushed red pepper. Set aside for now.

4.   Heat a large skillet using the medium temperature setting. Stir in the last 0.75 tbsp. of oil, shrimp and a pinch of sea salt. Cook for approximately 1.5 to 2 minutes per side.

5.   Push the shrimp to the side of the skillet. Whisk the eggs and spread into the open area of the skillet. Cook the eggs to a soft scramble (1 min.).

6.   Add the sauce mixture, noodles, cilantro, and green onions. Toss well. Heat until warmed.

7.   To finish, drizzle the rest of the lime juice over the skillet, and adjust the seasonings if desired.

8.   Garnish with crushed cashews and serve.

Nutrition: Proteins: 12 g Total Fat: 12 g Carbohydrates: 5 gCalorie Count: 180

Bacon Beef Pasta Time

Preparation Time: 5 minutes

Cooking time: 40–45 minutes

Servings: 8

Ingredients

- 1 pound extra-lean ground beef

- 8 slices center-cut bacon

- 1 large onion, chopped

- 2 cloves garlic, minced

- 3 cups mushrooms, quartered

- 2 (141/2-ounce) cans diced tomatoes, undrained

- 1 (24-ounce) jar pasta sauce

- 11/2 cups water

- 3 cups penne pasta

- 1 cup Colby & Monterey Jack cheeses, shredded

- 1/4 cup fresh parsley, chopped

Directions

1. Attach the bacon and cook over medium-high heat until crispy. Set aside, drain on paper towel and crumble.

2.   Clean the skillet and add the mushrooms, ground beef, onions and garlic.

3.   Stir-cook until lightly browned.

4.   Add half of the crumbled bacon on top; mix in the water, tomatoes, pasta and pasta sauce.

5.   Boil the mixture.

6.   Take the pasta mixture off the heat.

7.   Top with the remaining bacon and cheese.

8.   Set aside until the cheese melts and top with some parsley. Serve warm.

Nutrition: Calories 400 Fat 11 g Carbs 4.9 g Protein 25 g Sodium 570 mg

Tomato Kale Eggplant Skillet With Keto Linguine

Preparation Time: 12 minutes

Cooking Time: 30 minutes

Servings: 4

Ingredients:

- For the keto linguine:
- 1 cup shredded mozzarella cheese
- 1 egg yolk
- For the tomato-kale eggplant:
- 3 tbsp. olive oil
- 4 large eggplants, cut into 1-inch pieces
- Salt and black pepper to taste
- 1 yellow onion, chopped
- 4 garlic cloves, minced
- 1 cup cherry tomatoes, halved
- 1/2 cup vegetable broth
- 2 cups baby kale, chopped
- 1 cup grated parmesan cheese for serving
- 2 tbsp. pine nuts for topping

Directions:

1.   For the keto linguine:

2.   Pour the cheese into a medium safe-microwave bowl and melt in the microwave for 35 minutes or until melted.

3.   Take out the bowl and allow cooling for 1 minute only to warm the cheese but not cool completely. Mix in the egg yolk until well-combined.

4.   Lay a parchment paper on a flat surface, pour the cheese mixture on top and cover with another parchment paper.

5.   Place in a bowl and refrigerate overnight.

2.   When ready to cook, bring 2 cups of water to a boil in medium saucepan and add the keto linguine. Cook and then drain through a colander. Run cold water over the pasta and set aside to cool.

6.   For the tomato-kale eggplant:

7.   Heat the olive oil in a medium pot, season the eggplants with salt, black pepper, and sear in the oil until golden brown on the outside. Transfer to a plate and set aside.

8.   Attach the onion and garlic to the oil and cook until softened and fragrant, 3 minutes.

9.   Mix in the tomatoes and vegetable broth, cover and cook over low heat until the tomatoes soften and the liquid reduces by half. Season with salt and black pepper.

10.   Return the eggplants to the pot and stir in the kale. Allow wilting for 2 minutes.

11.   Divide the keto linguine onto serving plates, top with the kale sauce and then the parmesan cheese.

12.   Brush with the pine nuts and serve warm.

Nutrition: Calories: 442, Total Fat: 39.9g, Carbs: 1.5g, Fiber: 1g, Sugar: 2g, Protein: 7g

Sausage Fennel Pasta Meal

Preparation Time: 5 minutes

Cooking time: 15–20 minutes

Servings: 4–6

Ingredients

- 1 (141/2-ounce) can fire-roasted diced tomatoes

- 1/2 fennel bulb, thinly sliced

- 1 cup fresh basil leaves, torn

- 3/4 pound linguine

- 3/4 pound smoked Andouille sausage, cut into 1/2-inch

pieces

- 1 tablespoon kosher salt

- 1/2 teaspoon freshly ground pepper

- 2 tablespoons olive oil

- 41/2 cups water

Directions

1.   Add the oil to a large skillet or saucepan along with the tomatoes, pasta, basil, fennel, sausage, water, black pepper and salt.

2.   Stir and heat over medium-high heat.

3.   Allow the pasta mixture to boil gradually.

4.   Cook the mixture, stirring periodically, until the pasta is cooked to your satisfaction, about 8–9 minutes.

5.   Top with some basil and serve warm.

Nutrition: Calories 328 Fat 18 g Carbs 23 g Protein 10 g Sodium 985 mg

Creamy Tofu With Green Beans And Keto Fettuccine

Preparation Time: 40 minutes

Cooking Time: 60 minutes

Servings: 4

Ingredients:

- For the keto fettuccine:

- 1 cup shredded mozzarella cheese

- 1 egg yolk

- For the creamy tofu and green beans:

- 1 tbsp. olive oil

- 4 tofu, cut into thin strips

- Salt and black pepper to taste

- 1/2 cup green beans, chopped

- 1 lemon, zested and juiced

- 1/4 cup vegetable broth

- 1 cup plain yogurt

- 6 basil leaves, chopped

- 1 cup shaved parmesan cheese for topping

Directions:

1.   For the keto fettucine:

2.   Pour the cheese into a medium safe-microwave bowl and melt in the microwave for 35 minutes or until melted.

3.   Take out the bowl and allow cooling for 1 minute only to warm the cheese but not cool completely. Mix in the egg yolk until well-combined.

4.   Place in a bowl and refrigerate overnight.

5.   When ready to cook, bring 2 cups of water to a boil in medium saucepan and add the keto fettuccine. Cook and then drain through a colander. Run cold water over the pasta and set aside to cool.

6.   For the creamy tofu and green beans:

7.   Place the olive oil in a skillet, season the tofu with salt, black pepper, and cook in the oil until brown on the outside and slightly cooked through, 10 minutes.

8.   Mix in the green beans and cook until softened, 5 minutes.

9.   Stir in the lemon zest, lemon juice, and vegetable broth. Cook for 5 more minutes or until the liquid reduces by a quarter.

10.   Add the plain yogurt and mix well. Pour in the keto

fettuccine and basil, fold in well and cook for 1 minute.

11.   Dish the food onto serving plates, top with the

parmesan cheese and serve warm.

Nutrition: Calories: 721, Total Fat: 76.8g, Total Carbs: 2g,

Fiber: 0g, Sugar: 0g, Protein: 9g,

Pesto Parmesan Tempeh With Green Pasta

Preparation Time: 10 minutes

Cooking Time: 1 hour 27 minutes

Servings: 4

Ingredients:

- 4 tempeh

- Salt and black pepper to taste

- 1/2 cup basil pesto, olive oil-based

- 1 cup grated parmesan cheese

- 1 tbsp. butter

- 4 large turnips, Blade C, noodle trimmed

Directions:

1.   Preheat the oven.

2.   Season the tempeh with salt, black pepper and place on a baking sheet. Divide the pesto on top and spread well on the tempeh.

3.   Place the sheet in the oven and bake for 45 minutes to 1 hour or until cooked through.

4.   When ready, pull out the baking sheet and divide half of the parmesan cheese on top of the tempeh. Cook until the cheese melts. Remove the tempeh and set aside for serving.

5.   Melt the butter in a medium skillet and sauté the turnips until tender, 5 to 7 minutes. Stir in the remaining parmesan cheese and divide between serving plates.

6.   Top with the tempeh and serve warm.

Nutrition: Calories: 442, Total Fat: 29.4g, Saturated Fat: 11.3g, Total Carbs: 5g, Fiber: 1g, Sugar: 1g, Protein: 39g,

Wine Beef Pasta Meal

Preparation Time: 5 minutes

Cooking time: 30 minutes

Servings: 6

Ingredients

- 1 pound ground beef

- 1 stalk celery, chopped

- 3 cloves garlic, minced

- 1 large onion, chopped

- 1 medium carrot, chopped

- 1 teaspoon dried oregano or 1 tablespoon fresh oregano,

chopped

- 1 cup low-sodium beef broth

- 1/2 cup red wine

- 1 cup tomatoes, crushed

- 1/4 teaspoon ground black pepper (or to taste)

- 1/2 teaspoon salt (or to taste)

- 3 cups low-sodium vegetable broth

- 1 pound fettuccine or other pasta

- 2 tablespoons parsley, chopped (for garnish)

- Parmesan cheese, grated (for serving)

Directions

1. Add the beef to a large Dutch oven or deep saucepan and stir-cook over medium-high heat until lightly browned, about 5 minutes. Break into small pieces.

2. Add the onions, celery and carrot and sauté while stirring until softened, about 4–5 minutes.

3. Mix in the wine, garlic, oregano, tomatoes and beef broth. Season with salt and pepper.

4. Mix in the vegetable broth and pasta. Cook the mixture, stirring periodically, until the pasta is cooked to your satisfaction, about 18–20 minutes.

5. Take the pasta mixture off the heat.

6. Top with the Parmesan cheese and parsley; serve warm.

Nutrition: Calories 480 Fat 11 g Carbs 3 g Protein 27 g Sodium 871 mg

Mustard Tofu Shirataki

Preparation Time: 12 minutes

Cooking Time: 40 minutes

Servings: 4

Ingredients:

- For the shirataki angel hair:
- 2 (8 oz.) packs angel hair shirataki
- For the mustard sauce:
- 1 tbsp. olive oil
- 4 tofu, cut into strips
- Salt and black pepper to taste
- 1 medium yellow onion, finely sliced
- 1 medium yellow bell pepper, deseeded and thinly sliced
- 1 garlic clove, minced
- 1 tbsp. wholegrain mustard
- 5 tbsp. coconut cream
- 1 cup chopped mustard greens
- 1 tbsp. chopped parsley

Directions:

1. For the shirataki angel hair:

2.   Boil 2 cups of water in a medium pot over medium heat.

3.   Strain the shirataki pasta through a colander and rinse very well under hot running water.

4.   Allow proper draining and pour the shirataki pasta into the boiling water. Cook for 3 minutes and strain again.

5.   Place a dry skillet over medium heat and stir-fry the shirataki pasta until visibly dry, and makes a squeaky sound when stirred, 1 to 2 minutes. Take off the heat and set aside.

6.   For the mustard tofu sauce:

7.   Stir in the onion, bell pepper and cook until softened, 5 minutes.

8.   Mix in the mustard and coconut cream; simmer for 2 minutes and mix in the tofu and mustard greens. Allow wilting for 2 minutes and adjust the taste with salt and black pepper.

9.   Stir in the shirataki pasta, allow warming for 1 minute and dish the food onto serving plates.

10.   Garnish with the parsley and serve warm.

Nutrition: Calories: 375, Total Fat: 32.1g, Carbs: 5g, Fiber: 2gSugar: 4gProtein: 15g,

KETO CHAFFLE

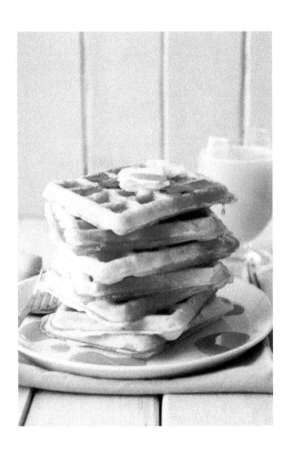

Fluffy Keto Chaffle: Wonder Bread Basic Chaffle

Preparation time: 5 minutes

Cooking time: 15 minutes

Servings: 2

Ingredients

- Almond flour (1 tbsp.)

- Water (1 tsp.)

- Keto-friendly mayo/sour cream (1 tbsp.)

- Baking powder (.125 tsp.)

- Egg (1)

- Pink Himalayan salt (1 pinch)

Directions:

1. Whisk each of the fixings in a mixing bowl.

2. Pour half of the batter into a waffle maker.

3. Prepare it until browned (3.5 to 4 min.).

Nutrition: Carbohydrates: 1.1 grams Calories: 134 Protein: 1.1 grams Fats: 11.6 grams

Onion Chaffle: Keto Copy-Cat Blooming Onion Chaffle Sticks & Dip

Preparation time: 5 minutes

Cooking time: 30 minutes

Servings: 2

Ingredients

- Eggs (2)

- Shredded part-skim mozzarella (4 oz.)

- Vidalia or sweet onion (Large slice/about 10 rings)

- Mayonnaise (2 tbsp.)

- Sugar-free ketchup (2 tsp.)

- Grated horseradish (1 tsp.)

- Smoked (.25 tsp.) OR Regular paprika (.25 tsp. + 5 drops of liquid smoke)

- Garlic powder (.125 tsp.)

- Onion powder (.125 tsp.)

- Dried oregano (.125 tsp.)

- Tabasco sauce/another hot sauce of choice (4-5 drops)

- Salt and pepper (as desired)

Directions:

1.   Preheat the Dash waffle maker.

2.   When waffle maker is hot, sprinkle with 0.5 ounces of the cheese

3.   Beat the eggs and pour 1/4 of the beaten egg over the cheese.

4.   Arrange 1/4 of the raw onion pieces over the cheese and egg.

5.   Sprinkle 0.5 ounces of cheese over the top. Close waffle maker and cook until top is crisp

6.   Remove the chaffle and cut it into strips.

7.   Repeat steps one through six to make four chaffles.

8.   Combine the dip fixings in a mixing bowl and whisk until smooth before serving.

Nutrition: Carbohydrates: 3 grams Calories: 163 Protein: 10 grams Fats: 12 grams

Chaffle & Chicken Lunch Plate

Preparation time 5 minutes

Cooking Time: 15 Minutes

Servings: 1

Ingredients:

- 1 large egg

- 1/2 cup jack cheese, shredded

- 1 pinch salt

- For Serving

- 1 chicken leg

- salt

- pepper

- 1 tsp. garlic, minutesced

- 1 egg

- I tsp avocado oil

Directions:

1.   Heat your square waffle maker and grease with cooking spray.

2.   Pour Chaffle batter intothe skillet and cook for about 3 minutesutes.

3.   Meanwhile,heat oil in a pan, over medium heat.

4.   Once the oil is hot, add chicken thigh and garlicthen,
cook for about 5 minutesutes. Flip and cook for another 3-4
minutesutes.

5.   Season with salt and pepper and give them a good mix.

6.   Transfer cooked thigh to plate.

7.   Fry the egg in the same pan for about 1-2 minutesutes
according to your choice.

8.   Once chaffles are cooked, serve with fried egg and
chicken thigh.

9.   Enjoy!

Nutrition: Protein: 31 Fat: 66 Carbohydrates: 2

Parmesan Garlic Chaffles

Preparation time: 5 minutes

Cooking time: 30 minutes

Servings: 1

Ingredients

- Shredded mozzarella cheese (.5 cup)

- Whole egg (1)

- Grated Parmesan cheese (.25 cup)

- Italian Seasoning (1 tsp.)

- Garlic powder (.25 tsp.)

Directions:

1. Heat the waffle iron and spritz it using coconut oil.

2. Whisk all of the fixings except for the mozzarella until combined. Then, add the cheese.

3. Add in half the batter to the center of the cooker. Close the lid and cook for three to five minutes, depending on how crispy you like the chaffles.

4. Serve with a spritz of oil, grated parmesan cheese, and freshly chopped parsley or basil to your liking.

Nutrition: Carbohydrates: 2 grams Calories: 352 Protein: 34 grams Fats: 24 grams

Grill Pork Chaffle Sandwich

Preparation time:

Cooking Time: 15 Minutes

Servings: 2

Ingredients:

- 1/2 cup mozzarella, shredded

- 1 egg

- I pinch garlic powder

- PORK PATTY

- 1/2 cup pork, minutesced

- 1 tbsp. green onion, diced

- 1/2 tsp Italian seasoning

- Lettuce leaves

Directions:

1.   Preheat the square waffle maker and grease with

2.   Mix together egg, cheese and garlic powder in a small mixing bowl.

3.   Pour batter in a preheated waffle maker and close the lid.

4.   Make 2 chaffles from thisbatter.

5. Cook chaffles for about 2-3 minutesutes until cooked through.

6. Meanwhile, mix together pork patty ingredients in a bowl and make 1 large patty.

7. Grill pork patty in a preheated grill for about 3-4 minutesutes per side until cooked through.

8. Arrange pork patty between two chaffles with lettuce leaves. Cut sandwich to make a triangular sandwich.

9. Enjoy!

Nutrition: Fat: 48 Carbohydrates: 4

Garlic Bread Chaffle

Preparation time: 5 minutes

Cooking time: 15 minutes

Servings: 2

Ingredients

- Large egg (1)

- Finely shredded mozzarella (.5 cup)

- Coconut flour (1 tsp.)

- Baking powder (.25 tsp.)

- Garlic powder (.5 tsp.)

- Butter - melted (1 tbsp.)

- Garlic salt (.25 tsp.)

- Parmesan (2 tbsp.)

- Minced parsley (1 tsp.)

Directions:

1. Set the mini waffle iron to preheat. Set the oven to 375° Fahrenheit.

2. Whisk/beat the egg, flour, baking powder, mozzarella, and garlic powder in a mixing bowl to combine.

3.   Pour half of the chaffle batter into the waffle iron and cook for three minutes or until the steam stops. Place the chaffle on a baking sheet.

4.   Repeat with the rest of the batter.

5.   Stir the butter and garlic salt to brush over the chaffles.

6.   Garnish the chaffles with parmesan.

7.   Bake for five minutes to melt the cheese. Sprinkle with parsley before serving.

Nutrition: Carbohydrates: 2 grams Calories: 186 Protein: 10 grams Fats: 14 grams

MAIN, SIDE & VEGETABLE

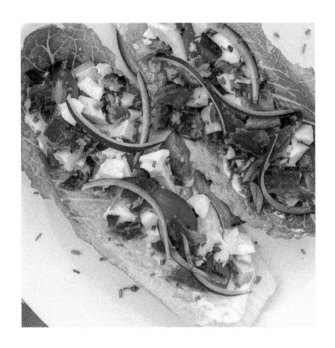

Peas Soup

Preparation time: 10 minutes

Cooking time: 10 minutes

Servings: 4

Ingredients:

- white onion, chopped
- tablespoon olive oil
- quart veggie stock
- eggs
- tablespoons lemon juice
- cups peas
- tablespoons parmesan, grated
- Salt and black pepper to the taste

Directions:

1. Heat up a pot with the oil over medium-high heat, add the onion and sauté for 4 minutes.

2. Add the rest of the ingredients except the eggs, bring to a simmer and cook for 4 minutes.

3. Add whisked eggs, stir the soup, cook for 2 minutes more, divide into bowls and serve.

Nutrition: Calories 293, fat 11.2 fiber 3.4, carbs 27, protein

4.45

Tamari Steak Salad

Preparation time: 15 minutes

Cooking time: 10 minutes

Servings: 2

Ingredients:

- large bunches salad greens

- 4 ounces beef steak

- ½ red bell pepper, diced

- 4 cherry tomatoes, cut into halves

- radishes, sliced

- tablespoons olive oil

- ¼ tablespoon fresh lemon juice

- 1-ounce gluten-free tamari sauce

- Salt as needed

Directions:

1. Marinate steak in tamari sauce.

2. Make the salad by adding bell pepper, tomatoes, radishes, salad green, oil, salt, and lemon juice to a bowl and toss them well.

3.   Grill the steak to your desired doneness and transfer steak on top of the salad platter.

4.   Let it sit for 1 minute and cut it crosswise.

5.   Serve and enjoy!

Nutrition: Calories: 500 Fat,: 37g Carbohydrates: 4g Protein: 33g Fiber: 2g Net Carbohydrates: 2g

Spinach Egg Muffins

Preparation time: 5 minutes

Cooking time: 10 minutes

Servings: 2

Ingredients:

- ½ cups chopped spinach
- 1/8 tsp dried basil
- 1/8 tsp garlic powder
- 2 large eggs
- 3 tbsp grated Parmesan cheese
- Seasoning:
- ¼ tsp of sea salt
- 1/8 tsp ground black pepper

Directions:

1.   Turn on the oven, then set it to 400 degrees F, and let preheat.

2.   Meanwhile, place eggs in a bowl, season with salt and black pepper and whisk until blended.

3.   Add garlic and basil, whisk in mixed and then stir in spinach and cheese until combined.

4.   Take two silicone muffin cups, grease them with reserved bacon greased, fill them evenly with prepared egg mixture and bake for 8 to 10 minutes until the top has nicely browned.

5.   Serve.

Nutrition: 55 Calories; 3.5 g Fats; 4.5 g Protein; 0.4 g Net Carb; 0.2 g Fiber;

Broccoli and Egg Muffin

Preparation time: 10 minutes

Cooking time: 10 minutes

Servings: 2

Ingredients:

- ¼ cup broccoli florets, steamed, chopped

- 2 tbsp grated cheddar cheese

- 1/16 tsp dried thyme

- 1/16 tsp garlic powder

- egg

- Seasoning:

- ¼ tsp salt

- 1/8 tsp ground black pepper

Directions:

1. Turn on the oven, then set it to 400 degrees F and let it preheat.

2. Meanwhile, take two silicone muffin cups, grease them with oil, and evenly fill them with broccoli and cheese.

3.   Crack the egg in a bowl, add garlic powder, thyme, salt, and black pepper, whisk well, then evenly pour the mixture into muffin cups and bake for 8 to 10 minutes until done.

4.   Serve.

Nutrition: 76 Calories; 5.1 g Fats; 5.7 g Protein; 1.2 g Net Carb; 0.7 g Fiber;

Acorn Squash Puree

Preparation Time: 10 minutes

Cooking Time: 20 minutes

Servings: 4

Ingredients:

- ½ cup water

- 2 acorn squash, deseeded and halved

- Salt and black pepper to the taste

- 2 tablespoons ghee, melted

- ½ teaspoon nutmeg, grated

Directions:

1. Put the squash halves and the water in a pot, bring to a simmer, cook for 20 minutes, drain, scrape squash flesh, transfer to a bowl, add salt, pepper, ghee and nutmeg, mash well, divide between plates and serve as a side dish.

Nutrition: Calories: 182 Fat: 3 Fiber: 2 Carbs: 7 Protein: 6

Amazing Carrots Side Dish

Preparation time: 10 minutes

Cooking time: 10 minutes

Servings: 12

Ingredients:

- 3 pounds carrots, peeled and cut into medium pieces
- A pinch of sea salt and black pepper
- ½ cup water
- ½ cup maple syrup
- 2 tablespoons olive oil
- ½ teaspoon orange rind, grated

Directions:

1. Put the oil in your instant pot, add the carrots and toss.

2. Add maple syrup, water, salt, pepper and orange rind, stir, cover and cook on High for 10 minutes.

3. Divide among plates and serve as a side dish.

4. Enjoy!

Nutrition: Calories 140, fat 2, fiber 1, carbs 2, protein 6

Butter Asparagus with Creamy Eggs

Preparation time: 5 minutes

Cooking time: 8 minutes

Servings: 2

Ingredients:

- 4 oz asparagus

- 2 eggs, blended

o oz grated parmesan cheese

- 1-ounce sour cream

- 2 tbsp butter, unsalted

- Seasoning:

- 1/3 tsp salt

- 1/8 tsp ground black pepper

- ¼ tsp cayenne pepper

- ½ tbsp avocado oil

Directions:

1. Take a medium skillet pan, place it over medium heat, add butter and when it melts, add blended eggs and then cook for 2 to 3 minutes until scrambled to the desired level; don't overcook.

2.   Spoon the scrambled eggs into a food processor, add 1/8 tsp salt, cayenne pepper, sour cream and cheese and then pulse for 1 minute until smooth.

3.   Return skillet pan over medium heat, add oil and when hot, add asparagus, season with black pepper and remaining salt, toss until mixed and cook for 3 minutes or more until roasted.

4.   Distribute asparagus between two plates, add egg mixture, and then serve.

Nutrition: 338 Calories; 28.5 g Fats; 14.4 g Protein; 4.7 g Net Carb; 1.2 g Fiber;

Fennel & Figs Lamb

Preparation time: 10 minutes

Cooking time: 40 minutes

Servings: 2

Ingredients:

- 6 ounces lamb racks

- fennel bulbs, sliced

- Salt

- pepper, to taste

- tablespoon olive oil

- figs, cut in half

- 1/8 cup apple cider vinegar

- 1/2 tablespoon swerve

Directions:

1. Take a bowl and add fennel, figs, vinegar, swerve, oil, and toss. Transfer to baking dish. Season with salt and pepper.

2. Bake it for 15 minutes at 400 degrees F.

3.   Season lamb with salt, pepper, and transfer to a heated pan over medium-high heat. Cook for a few minutes. Add lamb to the baking dish with fennel and bake for 20 minutes. Divide between plates and serve. Enjoy!

Nutrition: Calories: 230 Fat,: 3g Carbohydrates: 5g Protein: 10g Fiber: 2g Net Carbohydrates: 3g

Turkey and Cabbage Treat

Preparation Time: 5 minutes

Cooking time: 5 minutes

Servings: 4

Ingredients:

• tablespoon lard, at room temperature

• 1/2 cup onion, chopped

• pound ground turkey

• 10 ounces puréed tomatoes

• Sea salt and ground black pepper, to taste

• teaspoon cayenne pepper

• 1/4 teaspoon caraway seeds

• 1/4 teaspoon mustard seeds

• 1/2 pound cabbage, cut into wedges

• 4 garlic cloves, minced

• 1 cup chicken broth

• bay leaves

Directions:

1.	Press the "Sauté" button to heat up your Instant Pot. Then, melt the lard. Cook the onion until translucent and tender.

2.	Add ground turkey and cook until it is no longer pink; reserve the turkey/onion mixture.

3.	Mix puréed tomatoes with salt, black pepper, cayenne pepper, caraway seeds, and mustard seeds.

4.	Spritz the bottom and sides of the Instant Pot with a nonstick cooking spray. Then, place 1/2 of cabbage wedges on the bottom of your Instant Pot.

5.	Spread the meat mixture over the top of the cabbage. Add minced garlic. Add the remaining cabbage.

6.	Now, pour in the tomato mixture and chicken broth; lastly, add bay leaves.

7.	Secure the lid. Choose "Manual" mode and High pressure; cook for 5 minutes. Once cooking is complete, use a natural pressure release; carefully remove the lid.Bon appétit!

Nutrition: 247 Calories; 12.5g Fat; 6.2g Total Carbs; 25.3g Protein; 3.7g Sugars

SOUP AND STEWS

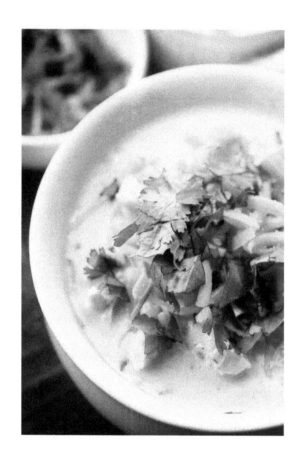

Creamy Broccoli Soup

Preparation time: 15 minutes

Cooking time: 4 hours

Servings: 7

Ingredients:

- 20 ounces (567 g) broccoli, cut into stalks and florets
- 3 tablespoons butter
- tablespoon olive oil
- red onion, roughly chopped
- garlic cloves, chopped
- pinch cayenne pepper
- ½ teaspoon paprika powder
- ½ teaspoon salt
- ¼ teaspoon ground black pepper
- cups chicken broth
- o ounces (99 g) Cheddar cheese, shredded
- ⅔ cup heavy whipping cream

Directions:

1.   Warm 1 tablespoon of butter and olive oil in a saucepan, then fry the broccoli stalks and chopped onion over medium heat for 5 minutes until tender.

2.   Put in the garlic and keep frying for 2 minutes until lightly browned, then sprinkle with cayenne pepper, paprika, salt, and ground black pepper. Cook for an additional 1 minutes.

3.   Pour over the chicken broth. Cover the lid and leave to simmer for 5 minutes.

4.   Remove the cooked vegetables from the saucepan to a food processor and process. Gently ladle the soup into the food processor while processing until creamy.

5.   Melt the remaining butter in the saucepan, and fry the broccoli florets for 5 minutes until soft and tender.

6.   Pour the soup from the food processor into the saucepan. Blend to mix well. If the soup is too thick, you can add some water to make it thinner.

7.   Bring the soup to a boil, then lower the heat and bring to a simmer over low heat for 3 minutes.

8.   Put in the Cheddar cheese and heavy whipping cream and cook for 2 minutes more until the cheese melts.

9.   Remove the soup from the saucepan and serve warm.

Nutrition: calories: 266 total fat: 23g net carbs: 7g fiber: 3g protein: 8g

Lemon Tahini Sauce

Preparation Time: 5 minutes

Cooking Time: 5 minutes

Servings: 2

Ingredients:

- 1/2 cup packed fresh herbs,(parsley, basil, mint, cilantro, dill, or chives)
- 1/4 cup tahini
- 1/4 cup of 1 Lemon Juice
- 1/2 teaspoon kosher salt
- tablespoon water

Directions:

1. Set everything in the bowl of a food processor fitted with the blade attachment or a blender. Process continuously until the herbs are finely minced, and the sauce is well-blended, 3 to 4 minutes.

2. Serve immediately or store in a covered container in the refrigerator until ready to serve.

Nutrition: Calories: 94 Fat: 8.1g Carbs: 4.3g Protein: 2.8g

Pumpkin And Sausage Soup

Preparation time: 5 minutes

Cooking time: 33 minutes

Servings: 4

Ingredients:

- ½ cup pumpkin puree

o   pounds (680 g) fresh sausage

- medium-sized red onion, minced

- small red bell pepper, diced

- ½ teaspoon red chili pepper flakes (optional)

- ½ teaspoon ground dried thyme

- ½ teaspoon dried sage

- garlic clove, minced

- 1 pinch salt

- cups chicken broth

- ½ cup heavy whipping cream

- tablespoons butter, melted

Directions:

1.   Sauté the sausage in a nonstick skillet over medium-high heat for 1 minutes, then add the onion and bell pepper.

Continue sautéing for 6 minutes until the sausage is lightly browned and the onion is translucent.

2. Fold in the chili pepper flakes, thyme, sage, minced garlic, and salt, then add the pumpkin puree, chicken broth, and heavy whipping cream.

3. Lower the heat and bring them to a simmer over low heat for 15 minutes or until thickened.

4. Pour the cooked soup into a large serving bowl and add the butter. Stir to mix well before serving.

Nutrition: calories: 777 total fat: 70g net carbs: 7g fiber: 2g protein: 27g

Almond Butter

Preparation Time: 15 minutes

Cooking Time: 15 minutes

Servings: 6

Ingredients:

- 2¼ cups raw almonds
- tablespoon coconut oil
- ¾ teaspoon salt
- 4-6 drops liquid stevia
- ½ teaspoon ground cinnamon

Directions:

1. Preheat the oven to 325 degrees F.

2. Arrange the almonds onto a rimmed baking sheet in an even layer.

3. Bake for about 12-15 minutes.

4. Remove the almonds from the oven and let them cool completely.

5. In a food processor, fitted with metal blade, place the almonds and pulse until a fine meal forms.

6.   Add the coconut oil, and salt and pulse for about 6-9 minutes.

7.   Add the stevia and cinnamon and pulse for about 1-2 minutes.

8.   You can preserve this almond butter in the refrigerator by placing it into an airtight container.

Nutrition: Calories: 226 Net Carbs: 3.2g Carbohydrate: 7.8g Fiber: 4.6g Protein: 7.6g Fat: 20.1g Sugar: 1.5g Sodium: 291mg

DESSERT

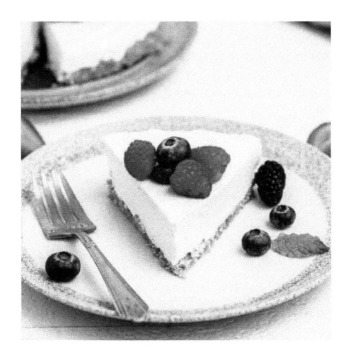

Keto Lemon Strawberry Cheesecake

Preparation Time: 15 minutes

Cooking Time: 0 minutes

Servings: 2

Ingredients:

- 2 pieces large strawberries

- 3 ounces cream cheese (softened)

- 2 teaspoons lemon extract

- 1/3 cup Swerve sweetener

- 3/4 cup heavy whipping cream

- zest of 1 lemon

Directions:

1. Prepare two 8-ounce mason jars.

2. In a mixing bowl, put in the whipping cream, sweetener, and cream cheese. Beat them on high setting until the texture becomes creamy and smooth.

3. Put in the lemon extract. Mix thoroughly.

4. Chop one of the strawberries into small pieces. The other strawberry should be sliced into thin heart-shaped slices.

5.   Fill each mason jar half-way with the cream cheese

mixture.

6.   Make a layer of chopped strawberries on top of the

cream cheese mixture in each jar.

7.   Fill the rest of each jar with the remaining cream cheese

mixture.

8.   Top each jar with the heart-shaped strawberry slices.

Arrange the slices to form a flower pattern.

9.   Sprinkle some lemon zest at the center of each flower.

10.   Put in the fridge to chill. Serve.

Nutrition: Calories: 474 Carbs: 5.7 g Fats: 48.2 g Proteins: 4.5

g Fiber: 0.4 g

Keto Gingerbread Spice Dutch Baby

Preparation Time: 12 minutes

Cooking Time: 30 minutes

Servings: 4

Ingredients:

- Heavy whipping cream 3/4 cup

- Eggs 5

- Cream cheese 2 oz.

- Vanilla extract 1 tsp.

- Maple extract 1/2 tsp.

- Powdered erythritol 1/3 cup

- Unflavored whey protein isolates 2 tbsp.

- Baking powder 1 tsp.

- Salt 1/4 tsp.

- Ground ginger 1 tsp.

- Ground cinnamon 1/2 tsp.

- Ground cloves 1/4 tsp.

- Unsalted butter for the pan 3 tbsp.

- Ground cinnamon

- Powdered erythritol, for dusting

- Heavy whipping cream, freshly whipped

Directions:

1. Preheat the oven to 400F

2. Place all ingredients, except for the butter, in a blender and blend until smooth and creamy. Blend for at least a minute to aerate the mixture. Set aside.

3. Put the butter in a 10-inch (25 cm) oven-proof skillet and place it in the oven. When the butter begins to sizzle, remove the pan from the oven, and pour the batter into the center of the hot skillet.

4. Bake for 12 to 15 minutes or until the Dutch baby is puffy and browned. The center should be just set. The Dutch baby is likely to rise in a lopsided fashion and will deflate somewhat as it cools.

5. Serve hot or cold. Garnish with a cinnamon dash, sprinkle of powdered sweetener, or a dollop of freshly whipped cream.

Nutrition: Calories 139 Total Fat 4.6 g Total Carbs 2.5 g Sugar 6.3 g Fiber 0.6 g Protein 3.8 g

Cocoa muffins

Preparation time: 10 minutes

Cooking time: 20 minutes

Servings 12

Ingredients:

- 1 1/4 Cups of Almond Flour
- 1/2 Cup of cocoa powder, unsweetened Cocoa Powder
- 1/2 cup of Erythritol
- 1 and 1/2 Teaspoons of Baking Powder
- 1 teaspoon of pure Vanilla Extract
- 3 Large eggs
- 2/3 Cup of heavy Cream
- 3 Ounces of melted almond butter
- 1/2 Cup of Chocolate Chips; Sugar-Free

Directions:

1.   Preheat your oven to a temperature of about 350 F.

2.   In a large bowl, combine the almond flour with the cocoa powder, the erythritol and the baking powder and mix very well

3.   Add in the vanilla extract, the eggs, and the heavy cream and mix very well.

4.   Add in the melted coconut oil and mix again

5.   Add in the sugar-free chocolate chips to your ingredients and stir very well.

6.   Line a muffin tray with cupcake papers

7.   Spoon your prepared mixture into the 12 holes of a standard muffin tray or any muffin tray you have

8.   Bake your muffins for about 20 minutes

9.   Remove the muffins from the oven and let cool for 5 minutes

10.   Serve and enjoy your delicious muffins!

Nutrition: Calories: 304 Fat: 23 g Carbohydrates: 4g Fiber: 2g Protein: 7

Flax Seed muffins

Preparation time: 8 minutes

Cooking time: 21 minutes

Servings 12

Ingredients:

- 1 Cup of ground golden flax seed

- 4 Large Pastured eggs

- 1/2 Cup of avocado oil or any type of oil

- 1/2 Cup of swerve

- 1/4 Cup of coconut flour

- 2 Teaspoons of vanilla extract

- 2 Teaspoons of cinnamon

- 1 Teaspoon of lemon juice

- 1/2 Teaspoon of baking soda

- 1 Pinch of sea salt

- 1 Cup of chopped walnuts

Directions:

1. Preheat your oven to a temperature of about 325 F.

2. If the flaxseed is not ground, grind it with a coffee grinder.

3. Mix the flax seeds with the pastured eggs, the avocado oil, the Swerve, the coconut flour, the vanilla extract, the cinnamon, the lemon juice, the baking soda, the salt and the walnuts with an electric mixer.

4. Prepare a muffin pan of 12 holes and line it with silicone muffin cups or parchment paper cups.

5. Distribute the batter evenly between the muffin cups; then bake it for about 18 to 21 minutes at a temperature of 325 F.

6. Serve and enjoy your muffins!

Nutrition: Calories: 218 Fat: 20g Carbohydrates: 5g Fiber: 3g Protein: 6.3

No Corn Cornbread

Preparation Time: 10 minutes

Cooking Time: 20 minutes

Servings: 8

Ingredients:

- 1/2 cup almond flour

- 1/4 cup coconut flour

- 1/4 tsp. salt

- 1/4 tsp. baking soda

- 3 eggs

- 1/4 cup unsalted butter

- 2 Tbsp. low-carb sweetener

- 1/2 cup coconut milk

Directions:

1. Preheat the oven to 325F

2. Combine dry ingredients in a bowl.

3. Put all the dry ingredients to the wet ones and blend well.

4. Dispense the batter into the baking pan and bake for 20 minutes.

5.   Cool, slice, and serve.

Nutrition: Calories: 65 Fat: 6g Carb: 2g Protein: 2g

Peanut butter muffins

Preparation time: 8 minutes

Cooking time: 21 minutes

Servings 12

Ingredients:

- 1 Cup of almond flour

- 1/2 Cup of So Nourished erythritol

- 1 Teaspoon of baking powder

- 1 Pinch of salt

- 1/3 Cup of peanut butter

- 1/3 Cup of almond milk

- 2 Large eggs

- 1/2 Cup of cacao nibs

Directions:

1.   Preheat your oven to a temperature of about 350 F.

2.   In a large mixing bowl; combine the almond flour with the baking powder, the salt and the erythritol.

3.   Add the peanut butter and the almond milk and stir.

4.   Add in the eggs, one at a time; then stir until each is fully whisked.

5.   Add in the cacao nibs and spray a muffin tin with cooking spray.

6.   Evenly distribute the batter between the muffin tins and bake for about 20 to 30 minutes.

7.   Remove the muffins from the oven and let cool for 5 minutes.

8.   Serve and enjoy your delicious muffins!

Nutrition: Calories: 265 Fat: 20.4g Carbohydrates: 4g Fiber: 2.7g Protein: 7.6g

Macadamia Cookies

Preparation time: 20 minutes

Cooking time: 10 minutes

Servings 11

Ingredients:

- 1/2 cup coconut oil, melted

- 2 tablespoons almond butter

- 1 egg

- 1 1/2 cup almond flour

- 2 tablespoons unsweetened cocoa powder

- 1/2 cup granulated erythritol sweetener

- 1 teaspoon vanilla extract

- 1/2 teaspoon baking soda

- 1/4 cup chopped macadamia nuts

- 1 Pinch of salt

Directions:

1.   Start by preheating your oven to a temperature of about 350 F.

2.   Combine the almond butter with the coconut oil, the almond flour, the cocoa powder, the swerve, the vanilla

extract, the baking soda, the chopped macadamia nut and the salt in a large mixing bowl.

3.   Mix your ingredients very well with a fork or a spoon; then set it aside.

4.   Line a cookie sheet with a parchment paper or just grease it very well.

5.   Drop small balls of about 1 1/2 inches wide; then gently flatten the cookies with your hands.

6.   Bake your cookies for about 15 minutes; then remove them from the oven and set them aside to cool for about 10 minutes.

7.   Serve and enjoy your cookies!

Nutrition: Calories: 179 Fat: 17 g Carbohydrates: 4g Fiber: 2g Protein: 5

Lightning Source UK Ltd.
Milton Keynes UK
UKHW020658210521
384116UK00005B/60

Healthy Ketogenic Diet Cookbook

A Completet Guide With Healthy and Easy Keto Diet Recipes To Weight Loss, Burn Fat And Live Better

Amelia Green